Code to Obesity:

Revealing the key to Achieving Weight Loss

By

Kurt D. Smith

TABLE OF CONTENTS

INTRODUCTION

We find ourselves in the middle of a magnificent tapestry of many studies that have sought to understand the underlying causes of obesity and effective remedies. As we proceed on an excursion into the maze of obesity research, we find ourselves in the heart of this complex tapestry. In spite of the tremendous quantity of knowledge that has been acquired over the course of human history, the riddle that surrounds the pandemic of obesity that occurred in the Western world around the year 1980 continues to remain obstinately elusive. Our notion of health has been challenged, and we have been pushed to hunt for remedies that have, up until this point, proven to be a mystery. This epidemic of fat, which is analogous to a silent tsunami, has spread across communities. This study takes on the immense work of unraveling the data, digging into the depths of research, and examining the numerous factors that may have ignited and propelled this unprecedented surge in obesity rates. This initiative comes at a time when the scientific community is striving to come to grips with a health concern that is both deep and increasing. The United States of America serves as the focal point of our inquiry, as it is the hub of this epidemic and the nation in which the reverberations of this health crisis resonate the most loudly. This pursuit is not merely an academic one; rather, it is a quest that has enormous repercussions for the health of the general public. We intend to accomplish our objective of gathering insights that can perhaps pave the way for prevention actions by evaluating the key variables that set the stage for the obesity epidemic. Not only can obesity have a detrimental influence on an individual's health, but it also has a huge impact on the well-being of society as a whole. It puts a demand on healthcare services and challenges our assumptions about what defines a healthy and thriving person. The stakes are enormous with obesity.

Throughout the entirety of our trip, we explore the currents of supposition that have surrounded the pandemic of obesity while simultaneously conceding that the cause behind the epidemic is still a mystery. Despite this, we are endowed with a multitude of research papers and an analytical lens, and we are working hard to discover patterns and linkages in order to acquire a deeper understanding of the causes that have led to the significant rise in obesity rates. In essence, this essay functions as a compass, directing us across the enormous landscape of obesity research and pushing us to handle the complexities of this multidimensional illness. As we dive into the depths of scientific inquiry, the objective is that our discoveries will not only cast light on the underlying causes of obesity but also identify avenues towards its prevention, delivering a beacon of insight in the continual struggle for world health and well-being.

CHAPTER ONE

THE OBESITY EPIDEMIC

The obesity pandemic emerged in the USA in 1976–1980 and subsequently expanded throughout Westernized nations. Many thousands of research studies have been done on the causes of obesity and successful measures of therapy. There has been considerable debate as to the real source of this pandemic, but, as of yet, no answer has achieved universal acceptance. The fact that the obesity pandemic didn't flash over nations like a wildfire—rather, it smoldered and then quietly increased year after year—has made it even more difficult to tackle because its causes have gotten so enmeshed into the social, environmental, and political fabric.

Regular surveys that assess the health and nutritional status of adults and children, known as the National Health and Nutrition Examination Survey (NHANES), are also carried out by the National Center for Health Statistics (NCHS), that is a part of the Centers for Disease Control and Prevention (CDC). Yet initiatives to tackle obesity largely through prevention are starting to gain momentum. To accomplish genuine advances, however, constructive change must come to all sections of society: governments and schools, companies and non-profit organizations, neighborhoods and communities, people, and families. We need to modify regulations and create an atmosphere where the default option is the healthy one. Obesity arises when energy intake (food) is much greater than energy expenditure (in particular, physical exercise).

What is obesity?

Obesity is a medical condition, often considered a disease, in which extra body fat has accumulated to such a degree that it might possibly have harmful consequences for health. It is a significant source of impairment and is connected with several illnesses and ailments, including cardiovascular diseases, diabetes, obstructive sleep apnea, some forms of cancer, and osteoarthritis. Body fat itself is not an illness, of course. But when your body has too much additional fat, it might affect the way it operates. These alterations are gradual, may worsen with time, and can lead to significant health repercussions. The good news is that you can improve your health risks by shedding some of your extra body fat. Not every weight-reduction approach works for everyone. Most individuals have attempted to lose weight more than once, and keeping the weight off is just as crucial as losing it in the first place. The reason is directly tied to changes in the American diet. There is a minimal connection between changes in the consumption of fat and carbohydrates.

This research gives the perspective that the element most directly associated with the pandemic is ultra-processed foods (UPFs) (i.e., meals with a high amount of calories, salt, sugar, and fat but with relatively few whole foods). Of particular concern is sugar consumption, particularly sugar-sweetened drinks (SSBs). There is considerable evidence that the use of SSBs leads to increased calorie intake and weight gain. A similar trend is also found with other UPFs. Factors that presumably contributed to the rising consumption of UPFs include their comparatively inexpensive price and the growing popularity of fast-food establishments. The reason for the obesity pandemic must thus be related to either an increase in energy intake from food or a reduction in physical activity (or a combination). As indicated above, it is doubtful that a decline in physical activity had a substantial influence on the outbreak. From this, we may deduce that the most plausible cause of the pandemic is changes in the American diet. A vast amount of data has connected diet with body weight and the danger of excess weight gain. A decline in physical activity appears to have had, at best, just a modest influence. Manual work has progressively declined in the USA over many decades. A considerable decline was recorded throughout the 1960s and 1970s, although this indicates only a modest link with the fast growth in obesity that occurred in the late 1970s.

Moreover, the extent of the drop in work-related physical activity is too minor to have a substantial influence on the rise in obesity. Finally, it is interesting that there is no data suggesting a reduction in leisure-time physical activity at approximately the time when the obesity epidemic began. Indeed, the late 1970s and 1980s were when exercise became increasingly popular (e.g., jogging). Many changes have taken place in the American diet during the last many decades. We now analyze how changes in the American diet may have contributed to the obesity pandemic. What are the kinds of obesity? Healthcare experts divide obesity into class categories depending on how severe it is using the BMI. If your BMI is between 25.0 and 29.0 kg/m2, they place you in the overweight group.

There are three broad types of obesity that healthcare experts use to determine what therapies may work best for each individual. These include:

- Class I Obesity: BMI 30 to<35 kg/m2
- Class II Obesity: BMI 35 to <40 kg/m2
- Class III Obesity: BMI 40+ kg/m2

CHAPTER TWO

THE POSSIBLE REASONS FOR THE EPIDEMIC

The reasons for obesity are as diverse as the individuals it affects. At its most basic, of course, obesity arises when someone routinely takes in more calories than required. The body stores these additional calories as body fat, and over time, the extra pounds build up. Eat less energy than the frame burns; weight goes down.

Below are the probable causes of obesity:

1) **Nutritional fats:** A concept that gained significant credence throughout the 1970s was that the meals typically consumed in the USA and across the Western world had an overly high level of fat and that this had a key impact on numerous chronic illnesses of the lifestyle. This theory was extended to obesity. In 1977, the Senate Select Committee on Nutrition and Human Needs converted this idea into real policy with the release of Dietary Goals for the United States. One of the suggestions in this study was that Americans should limit the fat level of their diet. This statement was reaffirmed in 1980 with the release of the first edition of Dietary Guidelines for Americans. Recommendations for a lower diet of fat slowly penetrated the general public. The food industry reacted by selling such goods as lean beef and low-fat milk. Despite these numerous initiatives, it is unclear whether there was a real

decline in fat consumption after 1980. Findings from NHANES surveys (of 8600–10,000 individuals) reveal that American adults lowered their fat consumption as a percentage of calories throughout the years 1976–1980 to 1999–2000 (36.7% to 32.3% in men; 36.0% to 32.4% in women). However, there was a large boost in calorie intake during the same period. The overall impact is that the amount of fat in the diet seems to have increased somewhat. Another study utilized information from the Nationwide Food Consumption Survey (NFCS) of 10,000 American individuals. The statistics span the period from 1977–1978 to 1987–1988. Fat consumption as a percentage of calories declined from 41.0% to 36.6%. There was also a moderate (about 4%) decline in calorie intake. The total outcome is an estimated 14% decline in the amount of fat in the diet. These data must be taken with some caution since they imply that calorie consumption is declining while the incidence of obesity is growing.

2) **Sugar and sugar-sweetened beverages:** Sugar consumption in the USA remained steady in the 1970s but then grew dramatically after 1978. Per capita consumption of total caloric sweeteners was 124.6 pounds in 1978, 132.7 pounds in 1988, and 154.1 pounds in 1997. This suggests an increase of 36.7 g/day (147 kcal/day) from 1978 and 1997. The rise in calorie consumption is sufficiently substantial to explain the increase in the average weight of the population. One crucial aspect that contributed to the surge in sugar consumption was

a huge decline in the price of sugar that happened after 1980. However, there was a substantial transition from sucrose to high-fructose corn syrup, although there is no firm evidence that this plays a significant role in the obesity epidemic. Also, the percentage of energy acquired from soft drinks grew from 4.1% to 7.0% at ages 19–39 and from 1.9% to 4.0% at ages 40–59. RCTs and prospective cohort studies have yielded solid evidence that the use of SSBs leads to increased calorie intake and weight gain. Findings from RCTs have revealed that the addition of SSBs to the diet of adults leads to a 0.85 kg rise in body weight.

Findings from cohort studies show that one additional serving per day of SSB is related to an increase in body weight in adults of roughly 0.12 to 0.22 kg. This is probably also true in the field of sugar consumption in general; however, there are significantly fewer research investigations. This research clearly implies that SSBs are a key factor responsible for the obesity pandemic.

3) **Ultra-Processed Foods:** SSBs are a kind of food frequently referred to as ultra-processed foods (UPFs). UPFs are often created using largely affordable sources of dietary energy and minerals, plus additives. They are generally heavy in calories, salt, sugar, and fat, yet they include limited quantities of entire foods. As a consequence, they have a low amount of dietary fiber, phytochemicals (for example, lutein, lycopene, and

anthocyanins), and other micronutrients, such as potassium, magnesium, and vitamin C. Examples of UPFs are white bread, sugary morning cereals, cookies, savory snacks, cakes, sweets, ice cream, margarine, sausages, and pizza. The results given here support the hypothesis that excessive amounts of UPFs in the diet have had a dominating role in the obesity pandemic. While the major emphasis here has been on the problem in the USA, it appears quite probable that UPFs are also strongly engaged in the pandemic of obesity that has swept throughout the Western world since about 1980. However, there are still significant gaps in the data, and much more study is consequently required. A high dietary intake of UPFs is strongly connected with a variety of harmful impacts on health, in addition to obesity. For that reason, dietary guidance should stress a decrease in the consumption of UPFs throughout the population. While health education, such as dietary guidelines and food labels, is a good way to strive towards that aim, many data points suggest this technique has very limited results. A more successful method is one based on rules and regulations imposed by governments. Examples of such measures include eliminating UPFs from school meals, raising the price of SSBs by imposing a tax, and utilizing subsidies to decrease the price of fruit and vegetables.

One aspect that may have been fueling the rising consumption of UPFs is the significant tendency toward dining at fast-food establishments. The studies of the American diet that were described previously indicated that the percentage of energy in the American diet that was received from dining out, including at fast-food restaurants, grew from 9.4% to 21.3% between the years 1977–1978 and 1994–1996. Fast-food restaurants may be of special concern since much of the food served there is UPF (e.g., burgers, fries, and cola beverages). Evidence from prospective cohort studies has revealed that more frequent dining at these restaurants is related to a larger rise in body weight. There is compelling evidence that UPFs have a substantial influence on the obesity pandemic. The above-mentioned studies of the American diet that reported a high growth in the consumption of SSBs over the period 1977–1978 to 1994–1996 also indicated a comparable increase in the intake of other UPFs. The highest increases were reported for salty snacks and pizza. During this time, the percentage of energy gained from different kinds of UPFs in the age range 40–59 grew from 1.4% to 3.8% for salty snacks, from 0.5% to 1.7% for pizza, from 0.5% to 1.4% for candy, and from 1.2% to 1.6% for French fries. There is a need to expressly underline the significance of decreasing the consumption of UPFs. Similarly, the addition of labels to the front of food containers may help buyers make better eating choices. Advising labels is one design that shows significant potential (e.g., advising customers that a product has a high concentration of sugar). Unfortunately, considerable studies clearly reveal that offering dietary advice to people has very little result. A far more successful technique is one based on laws adopted by governments that put rules on numerous entities, including the food industry. For example, schools may be instructed to stop selling UPFs at vending machines. Similarly, the number of UPFs in school meals should be decreased.

4) **The Impact of Farm Bills on the Cost of Food:** Analyses of food pricing have clearly revealed that better diets cost much more than less healthy diets. It is generally recognized that consumers prefer to purchase less expensive meals. As UPFs are a hallmark of less healthy meals, buyers will consequently commonly purchase these goods. These data clearly show, then, that relatively cheap food costs encourage the general public to consume UPFs, which, in turn, have a big impact on obesity. Manipulation of food prices is another policy technique that has tremendous promise. It is commonly documented that a rise in price leads to a fall in sales (and vice versa). This is known as price elasticity. Accordingly, taxes and subsidies may be employed in order to accomplish the desired impact on food consumption. In particular, the price of UPFs, especially sugar-rich foods, may be raised while the price of healthy foods, such as fruit, vegetables, and whole grains, can be cut. It is extremely plausible that policies adopted by governments are not only more successful than those focused on nutrition education, but they are also considerably more cost-efficient. This method has a lengthy history and has achieved considerable success. Prominent

examples include supplying people with clean drinking water, adding specific vitamins to particular meals, and eliminating trans fatty acids from foods.

It has been argued numerous times that a significant event contributing to the delivery of huge quantities of UPFs at relatively cheap costs was a major policy move by the Nixon government in the early 1970s. Farm bills established by the US Department of Agriculture (USDA) offered additional subsidies to farmers. This may have directly led to a big surge in the quantity of agricultural supplies that food producers subsequently transformed into UPFs, which were sold at a relatively cheap price.

5) **The impact of genetics on obesity**: Heredity has a role in obesity, but normally to a much smaller degree than many people may imagine. Rather than being obesity's primary cause, genes tend to raise the chance of weight gain and interact with other risk factors in the environment, such as bad diets and sedentary lifestyles. And healthy lives may mitigate these hereditary impacts. Within any given context, there is considerable diversity regarding body size and form among people. Part of this variety arises from genetic causes. To suggest that obesity might have a hereditary component is not unexpected, considering that it has been known for a long time that obesity commonly runs in families. Effectively, family research indicates that BMI is substantially connected with parental obesity. Children whose both parents are fat have an increased risk of becoming obese when compared with

children from non-obese parents. Nonetheless, in family research, it is difficult to differentiate whether this link originates from hereditary or environmental causes. This topic might be in part addressed by examining twin pairs or adopted children and giving data on genetic impacts on BMI. A meta-analysis of twin studies found that for adults, the BMI variance explained by genetic differences varied from 47% to 80%.

In accordance with these results, adoption studies provided evidence of the role of genetics in BMI. This research indicated that the BMI of adopted children correlated highly with biological parents and less with adoptive parents. Interestingly, certain genes implicated in producing fat in rodent models have also been identified as contributors to severe human obesity. Non-syndromic monogenic types of obesity come from mutations in a single gene and impact 5% of the population. These loss-of-function mutations are infrequent and often induce impairments in food intake and energy homoeostasis. The key portions of these mutations have been discovered in the LEP, leptin receptor (LEPR), melanocortin 4 receptor (MC4R), and pro-opiomelanocortin (POMC) genes. Interestingly, recent research discovered a deletion in the POMC gene with an allele frequency of 12% in Labrador retrievers, influencing their body weight and food desire, highlighting the relevance of the total leptin/melanocortin system on the obesity phenotype. Polygenic obesity is the most frequent kind of obesity in contemporary countries when the environment encourages weight gain owing to food availability and a lack of physical exercise. With the advent of technology and the completion of the Human Genome Project, our understanding of the genetic basis of obesity has expanded substantially in the past few years. Several studies emerged, finding more than 100 BMI-associated loci when comparing a sample comprised of normal-weight and obese people. The first locus obviously related to obesity, utilizing a genome-wide association (GWA) strategy, was the fat-mass and obesity-associated gene (FTO). Subsequent GWA research and meta-analysis found several variations related to common obesity. The most recent GWAS meta-analysis revealed 97 BMI-associated loci (56 of which were new) in research encompassing 339,224 European adults, contributing to 2.7% of BMI variance. It is still impossible to explain the fast development of obesity globally based merely on our genetic background. Understanding how genes impact systems of energy homoeostasis and generating variance in body weight within any given environment is vital. However, genes seldom have by themselves the capacity to define an individual's morphology, physiology, or behavior. It is the interplay between genes and the environment at all phases of the life cycle that may impact and trigger weight gain.

6) **The Influence of Prenatal and Postnatal Factors**: Early childhood is crucial too. Pregnant moms who smoke or who are overweight may have children who are more likely to grow up to be fat adults. Excessive weight gain during infancy

also boosts the chance of adult obesity, whereas being nursed may lessen the risk. Poorly designed diets What's become the standard Western diet—frequent, big meals loaded with refined carbohydrates, red meat, bad fats, and sugary drinks— plays one of the major roles in obesity. Foods that are absent in the Western diet—whole grains, vegetables, fruits, and nuts—tend to aid with weight management and also help avoid chronic illness. Studies have demonstrated a socioeconomic gradient in childhood obesity. Parental education as an indicator of socioeconomic status (SEP) had the most consistent, inverse connection with childhood obesity. Other SEP markers, such as parental occupation and family income, were more inconsistent.

In a meta-analysis, Wu and colleagues discovered that poor SEP is associated with a 10% greater risk of overweight and a 41% higher risk of obesity in children aged 0–15 years in high-income nations, especially in North America, Europe, and Oceania. Earlier studies on this topic presented results that showed that obesity is higher in people of low socioeconomic status in developed countries than in developing economies. 33 Socioeconomic factors are likely to be associated with child adiposity through a number of pathways, including knowledge, attitudes, financial constraints on nutrition, and physical activity patterns. Higher dangers of weight problems in kids with decrease SEP in advanced international locations can be associated with much less get admission to to wholesome meals and secure exercise, much less hobby in weight control, Cultural requirements of bodily effectiveness, and discrimination towards socioeconomic advancement. 34 However, a different picture can be found in developing countries and less economically developed areas, where malnutrition and opulence co-exist, food availability remains a daily challenge in populations with low SEP, and weight problems is finally perceived as a signal of wealth. Parental educational level is more consistently inversely linked with childhood obesity than other factors. As an essential socioeconomic indicator, parental educational level impacts the family's knowledge and ideas, and they are regarded as vital for healthy lifestyles and the development of obesity. Moreover, higher educational achievement may facilitate better understanding and utilization of available nutrition information that assists individuals' decisions on dietary practice, tend to follow recommendations for health behaviors, and respond more actively to health-related media messages than lower socioeconomic groups. Children from greater knowledgeable mother and father are much more likely to devour breakfast and eat fewer snacks, and they're much less in all likelihood to devour meals with excessive strength content, such as sweetened beverages, and more fruit and vegetable intake, contrary to children from low SES who tend to have diets rich in low-cost energy-dense foods, participate much less in bodily hobby sports, and feature decrease attention of weight control. The place where families dwell might also lead to a less healthy eating regimen. Children living in more poor locations tend to consume fewer fruits and vegetables but more sugar and sweets, fatty processed meats, salty snacks, and soft beverages compared with those from better-income homes. Excessive food consumption is a primary factor in obesity.

Another big cause of obesity is the absence of physical exercise and sedentary behavior assessed by screen time. Sallis and colleagues identified a socioeconomic gradient in sedentary behavior, physical activity, and access to physical activity facilities among young people. Families residing in poverty have one-of-a-kind priorities than people with a solid SEP. Those confronting poverty are more susceptible to experiencing disinvestment in health and healthful activities. The socioeconomic gradient in childhood obesity in certain communities may partially be attributable to a healthy diet and physical exercise being deemed a low priority in disadvantaged homes. This dilemma is even more difficult when we adopt a contextual picture of our environment.

Modern eating environments are loaded with nutrient-poor and energy-dense meals. These meals are very tasty and prepared in ways that make it challenging for the body to manage consumption and weight. This inherent sensitivity to ultra-processed meals is particularly troublesome for youngsters since they have a larger taste for sweet foods than adults. Childhood is a phase in a person's life when companies try to create brand loyalty. Marketing and early exposure at a young age to ultra-processed meals affect children's taste expectations and preferences for harmful items. Too much time spent watching television, not enough physical activity, and not enough sleep Television viewing is a substantial obesity risk factor, in part because exposure to food and beverage advertising might affect what individuals consume. Physical movement helps guard against weight gain, but internationally, people simply aren't doing enough of it. Lack of sleep—another feature of the Western lifestyle—is increasingly emerging as a risk factor for obesity. hazardous environment—food and physical activity Several writers claim that the worldwide growth of obesity is being driven mostly by environmental factors such as excessive food intake, high-sugar drinks, less exercise, television viewing, etc. rather than biological ones. Nowadays, as a consequence of social globalization, we are daily exposed to pictures and offers of high-fat, calorie-dense, delicious, and economical meals. Furthermore, our physical needs have altered, resulting in an imbalance in energy intake and expenditure. The contemporary lifestyle forces humans to live in an obesogenic environment, pushing us to eat more and exercise less. For example, multiple research projects identified a link between obesity and time spent watching television in both adults and children. From an evolutionary standpoint, it is entirely the opposite of the period when people were more active and had constraints on food consumption. Several assessments of obesity refer to the possible role of environmental variables that encourage excessive food intake and inhibit physical exercise. Recently, there has been a rising acknowledgment of socioeconomic issues leading to obesity.

Regarding, for example, children, numerous causes have been identified to explain the contemporary pandemic of juvenile obesity. However, the mechanisms of childhood obesity are exceedingly complicated and remain unknown. Obesity exhibits complex interactions among genetic, metabolic, behavioral, cultural, and environmental variables. The bulk of the studies depend on child and parent traits and have not explored the family system or the multilayered environment in which child risk factors originate. It is crucial to evaluate both biological and social causes of childhood obesity at three levels (individual, family, and community) and throughout early life. Among the various variables that cause juvenile obesity, parental and family histories of obesity may have major impacts via genetic as well as environmental factors. Family variables have a large impact since family members are likely to have similar diets, screen time, and physical activity behaviors, as well as a major effect of beliefs and attitudes surrounding food and exercise that leads to obesity. As crucial as individual decisions are when it comes to health, no one person operates in a vacuum. The physical and social environment in which individuals live has a big effect on the diet and exercise choices they make. And, sadly, in the U.S. and increasingly throughout the world, this atmosphere has become poisonous to healthy living. The relentless and inescapable promotion of unhealthy foods and sugary beverages. The absence of safe spaces for exercise. The junk food is sold at school, at work, and at the neighborhood shop. Add it all up, and it's harder for folks to make the healthy choices that are so vital to a decent quality of life and a healthy weight. Another factor that recently surfaced as accounting for obesity development is the gut microbiota, which contains a diverse colony of bacteria residing in the human gastrointestinal tract. Several pieces of evidence imply that nutrition changes gut flora, and this is mirrored by variations identified between obese and lean people.

Furthermore, numerous investigations have pointed to the relevance of gut bacteria in controlling calorie intake. The importance of epigenetic profiles and gut microbiota in obesity is far more nuanced than this quick summary. Indeed, there is rising evidence from various research and reviews that shows the role of these players in obesity. Nevertheless, additional controlled and standardized investigations are required to access the true influence of these players on obesity. Obesity prevention approaches:

Turning Around the Epidemic

Evidence demonstrates that obesity prevention policy and environmental change initiatives should concentrate on enabling a number of critical behaviors. This area of the website presents potential measures for obesity prevention based on a study of expert advice from key governmental, professional, and public health advocacy groups. Inside, you will discover high-level suggestions for improvements in key settings—families, early childcare, schools, worksites, healthcare organizations—and for broad, community-wide adjustments in the food and activity environments that may help make healthy choices simpler choices for everyone. Each page also contains connections to toolkits, guidelines, and other relevant resources for putting these obesity prevention techniques into practice. Over time, we will add more obesity prevention techniques, guidelines, and resources as more research arises. Keep in thoughts that those weight problems prevention hints are primarily based totally typically on an assessment of U.S. expert guidance, unless otherwise indicated; in other countries, different policy approaches may be needed to achieve improvements in food and physical activity environments, including choosing healthier foods (whole grains, fruits and vegetables, healthy fats, and protein sources) and beverages. • Limiting unhealthy meals (refined grains and sweets, potatoes, red meat, processed meat) and beverages (sugary drinks) • Increasing physical activity • Limiting television time, screen time, and other "sit time" • Improving sleep • Reducing stress

CHAPTER THREE

WAYS TO SAVE A LOT OF CALORIES

There are simple yet extremely efficient techniques to limit calories and lose weight. To lose weight, you need to eat fewer strength than you burn. However, limiting the quantity of food you consume to minimize calories might be tough.

Count your calories: One technique to make sure you don't consume too many calories is to count them. In the past, recording calories was fairly time-consuming. However, current applications have made it faster and simpler than ever to monitor what you consume. Some applications also give daily lifestyle recommendations to help keep you engaged. This may be more beneficial than merely tracking your consumption, since it might help you build good, long-term habits.

Use less sauce: Adding ketchup or mayonnaise to your dish might contribute more calories than you anticipate. In fact, merely 1 tablespoon (15 ml) of mayonnaise provides an additional 57 calories for your meal. If you use a lot of sauce, consider eating a little less, or not using it at all, to lower the amount of calories you're consuming.

Don't drink your calories: Drinks may be a neglected source of calories in your diet. Sugar-sweetened beverages, such as soda, are also connected to obesity and type 2 diabetes. A single 16-ounce (475-ml) bottle of Coke has approximately 200 calories and 44 grams of sugar. Research reveals that consuming a lot of sugar-sweetened drinks not only adds many unneeded calories to your diet but may also increase your appetite later on. You may want to cut down on other high-sugar, high-calorie beverages as well. These include alcohol, certain commercially made coffee drinks, and sugar-sweetened fruit juices and smoothies.

Don't add sugar to tea and coffee: Tea and coffee are nutritious, low-calorie liquids, but spooning in only 1 teaspoon (4 grams) of sugar adds roughly 16 calories to your cup. Though this may not seem like much, the calories in a few cups or glasses of sugar-sweetened tea a day may mount up.

Cook your own food: When you purchase food cooked by someone else, you don't always know what's in it. Even meals you assume are healthy or low-calorie might have hidden carbohydrates and fats, driving up their calorie value. Cooking your own meals gives you more control over the quantity of calories you ingest.

Don't keep junk food in the home: If you put junk food within easy reach, it's much simpler to consume. It might be particularly troublesome if you tend to eat when you're worried or bored. To avoid the impulse to go for unhealthy foods, keep them out of the house.

Use smaller plates: Today's dinner plates are, on average, 44% bigger than they were in the 1980s. Greater plates have been associated with greater serving sizes, which suggests individuals are more likely to overeat. In one instance, research indicated that participants using bigger dinner plates at a buffet ate 45% more food than those who utilized the smaller plate size. Choosing a smaller plate is a simple strategy that might keep your portion proportions on track and reduce overeating.

Bulk-up dishes with veggies: Most people don't consume enough vegetables. In fact, it's estimated that roughly 87% of individuals in the United States don't consume the required amount. Filling half your plate with veggies is a fantastic method to enhance your vegetable consumption while cutting down on higher-calorie meals.

Drink water before your meal: Drinking water before a meal may help you feel more content, leading you to consume fewer calories. As an example, one study revealed that drinking only 2 cups (500 ml) of water before a meal cut calorie consumption by roughly 13%. It may assist you lose weight.

Have a low-calorie starting: Studies suggest that picking a low-calorie appetizer, such as a light soup or salad, may prevent you from overeating. In fact, research has discovered that having soup before a large meal might cut the overall amount of calories you consume by as much as 20%.

Eat your meals slowly: Taking your time with a meal and chewing slowly may help you feel full more quickly, which might help you eat less. If you're prone to eating in haste, consider putting your knife and fork down between mouthfuls or counting the number of times you chew your meal.

Order high-calorie dressings on the side: Sometimes even healthful, low-calorie meals like salads may be surprisingly heavy in calories. This is particularly true when a salad arrives with a huge quantity of high-calorie dressing poured over it. If you want a dressing on your salad, request it on the side so you can manage how much you're using.

Watch your portion amount: Confronted with enormous quantities of food, individuals are more likely to overeat. This is one dilemma individuals confront at all-you-can-eat buffets, where it's easy to consume considerably more than you expected. To prevent overeating, you might try weighing and measuring your meals or using smaller dishes, as mentioned above.

Eat without distractions: Your environment has a big effect on how much you eat from day to day. Studies suggest that if you're preoccupied when you eat, you're far more likely to overeat, even at later meals. For example, one recent assessment indicated that people who were preoccupied during dining ingested 30% more snacks than those who were conscious of their meal. Unhealthy distractions include watching TV, reading a book, using your cell phone, or sitting at your computer while eating.

Don't clean your plate: Most individuals are conditioned to consume whatever is placed in front of them. Still, you don't need to consume all the food on your plate if you're not hungry. Instead, try eating thoughtfully. This is eating with attention to what you're doing and how you feel. With this knowledge, you can eat simply until you're satisfied, not until you've cleared your plate.

Eat smaller versions of sweets and desserts: Many popular brands of ice cream and chocolate come in small- as well as full-size varieties. If you want a sweet treat, selecting a smaller size of your favorite dessert might give you the fix you want and save you a lot of calories. If you're dining out, minimize your portion by splitting your dessert with a companion.

Take half home while dining out: Restaurants typically provide large quantities that include much more calories than you need in one sitting. To prevent eating too much, ask your waitress to wrap up half of your meal before they serve it so you can take it home. Alternatively, you may percentage it with a friend. One study indicated that people who successfully sustained weight reduction typically shared meals or ordered half-servings when they ate out.

Eat with your non-dominant hand: This may seem a bit odd, but if you're prone to eating rapidly, eating with your non-dominant hand might be useful. It will sluggish you down, so that you devour less.

Include protein with every meal: Eating additional protein is regarded as a beneficial technique for weight reduction and maintenance. One explanation for this is that protein may fill you up more than other foods, and feeling full might stop you from overeating. To gain these advantages, consider including a high-protein item in most of your meals.

Don't touch the bread basket: When you're hungry, it's easy to grab the pre-dinner snacks at a restaurant. However, this practice may add hundreds of calories to your meal, particularly if you're nibbling bits of bread and butter. Send the bread basket back to avoid consuming a lot of calories before your main meal comes.

Order two appetizers: Overly huge amounts are a main factor in individuals overeating. If you're dining out and know a restaurant provides enormous amounts, you may order two appetizers instead of an appetizer and a main course. This way, you can enjoy two dishes without overdoing it.

Make healthy substitutions: One technique to reduce a few calories is to adjust the food you have selected to consume. For example, if you're eating a burger, leaving out the bread will save you roughly 160 calories—or even more if the bun is extremely huge. You can even cut a few calories off your sandwich by eliminating one layer of bread to build your own open-faced sandwich, even if it's not on the menu. What's more, replacing fries or potatoes with more veggies can enhance your vegetable consumption while cutting down on calories.

Choose lower-calorie alcoholic drinks: Many individuals are cautious about what they eat throughout the week but then binge drink on weekends. Choose clean alcohol with a low-calorie mixer over beer, wine, or a cocktail. This will help you avoid extra calories from the beverages.

Don't go big: Sometimes, buying a bigger drink or side for just a tiny increase in price may seem like a better value. However, most restaurants already provide enormous food and drink quantities, so stick to the standard size.

Skip the extra cheese: Extra cheese is sometimes an option at restaurants. Still, even a single slice of cheese may contribute about 100 calories to your dinner.

Change your cooking techniques: Cooking your own meals is a terrific way to keep your meals nutritious and your calorie consumption under control. Nonetheless, certain cooking techniques are preferable to others if you're attempting to cut down on calories. Grilling, air-frying, steaming, stewing, boiling, or poaching are healthier choices than frying in oil.

Choose tomato-based sauces instead of creamy ones: Creamy sauces not only contain more calories but frequently also include fewer veggies. If you have an option, consider a tomato-based sauce over a creamy one to receive the double advantage of fewer calories and more healthful veggies.

Learn to read food labels: Not all convenience foods are bad, but many include hidden fats and carbohydrates. It's much simpler to find healthy selections if you know how to read food labels. You should also examine the serving size and quantity of calories, so you know how many calories you're actually ingesting.

Eat whole fruits: Whole fruits carry fiber, vitamins, minerals, and antioxidants, making them a wonderful complement to your diet. Additionally, compared to fruit juice, fruits are harder to overeat since they fill you up. Whenever feasible, select whole fruits over fruit juice. They're more satisfying and offer more nutrients with fewer calories.

Dip veggies, not chips: If you prefer eating snacks, such as chips and dips, while watching TV but want to cut down on calories, just go for nutritious veggies instead.

Don't consume animal skin: Eating the skin on your meat adds additional calories to your meal. For example, a skinless roasted chicken breast is roughly 142 calories. The identical breast with skin has 193 calories.

Skip the second serving: If a meal is great, you may be inclined to go back for more. However, engaging in a second helping might make it harder to estimate how much you've eaten, which may make you ingest more than you meant. Go for a moderately big piece the first time and skip seconds.

Choose a thin crust: Pizza is a popular quick dish that may be quite high in calories. If you want to eat some pizza, keep the calories to a minimum by picking a thinner crust and lower-calorie toppings, such as veggies.

Try intermittent fasting: Intermittent fasting is a popular weight-reduction approach that may help you decrease calories. This strategy of dieting works by cycling your eating habits between times of fasting and eating. It's particularly helpful for weight reduction since it makes it simpler to lower the quantity of calories you consume over time. There are many various methods to conduct intermittent fasting, so it's simple to discover a strategy that works for you.

Get adequate sleep: Lack of sleep has been linked to obesity. In fact, those who don't sleep well tend to weigh more than those who are routinely well rested. One explanation is that sleepless people are more likely to feel hungry and consume more calories. If you're attempting to limit calories and lose weight, make sure you routinely get a decent night's sleep.

Overfed yet undernourished—how is this possible?

One of the reasons why it may be a tough topic to comprehend is because our knowledge and comprehension of calories are restricted. Nutritional science has long portrayed that all calories are created equal, and with the correct quantity of caloric intake, we should obtain all the nutrients we need; hence, it would be impossible to be malnourished. However, there is mounting evidence to show a calorie is not simply a calorie, and the sooner we move away from the limited perspective of energy intake and expenditure, the better we grasp the intricacies of nutrition and obesity. The quality of calories is also crucial, and we should be urging people to examine the additional nutritive value of foods (saturated fat, protein, fiber, or vitamin C) when selecting food and drink, not simply the calorie intake. Unfortunately, the normal Western diet is low in fresh fruits, vegetables, and whole grains but contains high quantities of refined, processed, and sugary foods. The latter are often heavy in calories (or empty calories, as many call them) and not much else, therefore commonly referred to as an 'energy dense (high in calories) and nutrient poor (low in nutritional value) diet. Energy-dense meals are often heavy in fat (e.g., butter, oils, fried foods), sugars, or carbohydrates, whereas energy-dilute foods have a high water content (e.g., fruits and vegetables). We know that a high consumption of energy-dense meals promotes weight gain and that the probability is that these items are routinely eaten by the overweight and obese population. These diets are also often white, processed items like white bread or pasta, which have had the fiber removed during processing, along with iron and many critical B vitamins, to provide a more pleasant flavor and texture that the 21st century is so used to. Combined with poor consumption of fiber-rich fruits and vegetables, it is of little surprise that the UK's fiber consumption is exceptionally low—adults and children consume much less than the recommended intake of 30 g/day. Fibre is an incredibly important nutrient and can help to prevent bowel cancer, protect against high cholesterol, and reduce the risk of type 2 diabetes. Fibre has a low glycaemic index (GI), which means fiber-rich foods allow the slow release of sugars into our body and therefore prevent blood sugar spikes, keep us fuller for longer, and therefore make us less likely to have additional snacks throughout the day.

Why are we consuming these kinds of foods?

High-calorie, processed meals are reported to be cheaper than healthy, fresh, high-quality meat, fruit, and vegetables; however, this is widely challenged by numerous stakeholders. Other variables that may explain the rising consumption of these meals are that they frequently require less preparation, which is crucial for customers searching for convenience in busy working lives and also for people who have weak food preparation abilities. However, with the majority of the population becoming overweight or obese in the UK, we have to go beyond individual decisions in our diet and evaluate what is going on around us and how this may be impacting what we eat. Millions of pounds of money is put into the marketing of unhealthy food and drink in the UK every year. The industry doesn't spend this amount of money merely for fun. There is compelling evidence to indicate exposure to advertising for unhealthy food and drink might alter our tastes, consumption patterns, and weight status. In addition to this, consumption of sugar-sweetened beverages, living sedentary lifestyles, promotions on unhealthy food and drink products, and other environmental influences play a key role in the growing trend of obesity, increasing the likelihood of consuming energy-dense, nutrient-poor diets, which could lead to deficiencies in essential vitamins and minerals. On a more positive note, this expanding body of data reveals a possible additional advantage of lowering obesity in that it may help decrease the incidence of nutritional inadequacies in the population. Policymakers and public health should examine the possible nutritional inadequacies of the obese population while delivering primary care and treatment, as well as initiatives to avoid obesity and nutritional deficiencies in the future.

CHAPTER FOUR

TIPS FOR SUCCESSFUL WEIGHT LOSS

Successful weight reduction does not require individuals to follow a particular diet plan, such as Slimming World or Atkins. Instead, they should concentrate on consuming fewer calories and exercising more to establish a negative energy balance. Weight reduction is mostly based on lowering the overall consumption of calories, not altering the quantities of carbohydrate, fat, and protein in the diet. An acceptable weight loss target to start experiencing health benefits is a 5–10 percent decrease in body weight over a 6-month time period. Most individuals may reach this aim by lowering their overall calorie consumption to somewhere in the range of 1,000–1,600 calories per day. A diet of less than 1,000 calories per day will not provide the necessary daily sustenance. People who have a BMI equal to or greater than 30 and no obesity-related health concerns may benefit from using prescription weight-loss drugs. These could also be helpful for those with a BMI equal to or greater than 27 with obesity-related illnesses. However, a person should only utilize drugs to assist in the aforesaid lifestyle improvements. If efforts to reduce weight are unsuccessful and a person's BMI reaches 40 or more, surgical treatment is a possibility.

Maintaining weight loss involves a commitment to a healthy lifestyle, from which there is no "vacation." Although people should feel free to enjoy a special meal out, a birthday celebration, or a joyful holiday feast without feeling guilty, they should try not to stray too far from the path of healthy eating and frequent physical activity. Those who do may discover that they lose concentration. Gaining back lost weight is simpler than losing it. Achieving and sustaining weight reduction is attainable when individuals make lifestyle modifications in the long term. Regardless of any particular ways that assist a person in losing weight, people who are cognizant of how and what they eat and participate in daily physical activity or regular exercise will be effective both in losing and keeping off extra weight. A balanced lifestyle and healthy food are the keys to healthier living and improved weight management. Some ideas for weight reduction include exercising frequently, obtaining social support, and maintaining a diet and weight diary. According to the Centers for Disease Control and Prevention, roughly 93.3 million individuals in the United States had obesity in 2015–2016. This amount is comparable to 39.8 percent of the population. Carrying extra body weight may raise the risk of major health issues, including heart disease, hypertension, and type 2 diabetes. Crash diets are not a sustainable option, whatever rewards their proponents may claim they offer. To both lose weight safely and maintain that weight reduction over time, it is vital to undertake gradual, persistent, and positive lifestyle adjustments.

In this post, we present 10 strategies for weight management. People may reduce weight and sustain this decrease by completing numerous manageable actions. These include the following:

1. Eat variety, colorful, nutritionally packed meals: Healthful food and snacks have to represent the cornerstone of the human diet. An easy method to develop a meal plan is to make sure that each meal consists of 50 percent fruit and vegetables, 25 percent healthy grains, and 25 percent protein. Total fiber consumption should be 25–30 grams daily. Eliminate trans fats from the diet and reduce the consumption of saturated fats, which has a significant relationship with the occurrence of coronary heart disease. Instead, individuals may ingest monounsaturated fatty acids (MUFA) or polyunsaturated fatty acids (PUFA), which are kinds of unsaturated fat. The following foods are nutritious and generally high in nutrients:

• Fresh fruits and veggies

• Fish

• Legumes

• Nuts

• Seeds

• Whole grains, such as brown rice and oats

• Foods to avoid eating include:

• Foods with additional oils, butter, and sugar

• Fatty red or processed meats

• Baked goods

• Bagels

• White bread

Processed foods In rare situations, omitting specific items from the diet could lead a person to become deficient in some important vitamins and minerals. A nutritionist, dietitian, or other healthcare expert may advise a person on how to consume adequate nutrients while pursuing a weight reduction program.

2. Keep a food and weight diary: Self-monitoring is a vital aspect of effectively reducing weight. People can use a paper diary, cellular app, or committed internet site to document each object of meals that they devour every day. They may also monitor their success by noting their weight on a weekly basis. Those who can measure their performance in modest increments and observe bodily improvements are considerably more likely to adhere to a weight reduction strategy. People may also keep track of their body mass index (BMI) by utilizing a BMI calculator.

3. Engage in frequent physical activity and exercise: Regular workout is important for each bodily and intellectual health. Increasing the frequency of bodily pastime in a disciplined and practical manner is frequently important for a success weight loss. One hour of moderate-depth hobby in line with day, consisting of brisk walking, is ideal. If one hour in line with day isn't possible, the Mayo Clinic shows that someone must goal for no less than a hundred and fifty mins each week. People who aren't commonly bodily energetic ought to slowly boom the quantity of workout that they do and regularly boom its intensity. This approach is the most sustainable way to ensure that regular exercise becomes a part of their lifestyle. In the same way that logging meals might psychologically aid with weight reduction, individuals may also benefit from keeping track of their physical activity. Many free smartphone applications are available that measure a person's calorie balance once they register their food consumption and activity. If the notion of a complete workout sounds frightening to someone who is new to exercise, they might begin by undertaking the following exercises to raise their activity levels:

• Taking the stairs

• Raking leaves

• Walking a dog

• Gardening

• Dancing

• Playing outdoor games

• Parking further away from a building entrance.

Individuals who have a minimal risk of coronary heart disease are unlikely to need a medical examination prior to commencing an exercise plan. However, a previous medical examination may be necessary for certain patients, especially those with diabetes. Anyone who is unclear about acceptable amounts of exercise should talk to a healthcare practitioner.

4. Eliminate liquid calories: It is possible to ingest masses of energy an afternoon via way of means of ingesting sugar-sweetened soda, tea, juice, or alcohol. These are characterized as "empty calories" because they provide greater energy content without delivering any nutritional advantages. Unless a person is having a smoothie to substitute for a meal, they should attempt to stick to water or unsweetened tea and coffee. Adding a dash of fresh lemon or orange to water may enhance taste. Avoid confusing dehydration with hunger. A person may typically satisfy sensations of hunger between planned meal times with a glass of water.

5. Measure servings and manage portions: Eating too much of any meal, including low-calorie veggies, may result in weight gain. Therefore, consumers should avoid calculating portion sizes or consuming food right from the package. It is recommended to use measuring cups and serving size recommendations. Guessing results in overestimating and the opportunity of eating a larger-than-vital meal. The following size comparisons might be beneficial for tracking meal consumption while eating out:

• A quarter of a cup is a golf ball.

• One-half of a cup is a tennis ball.

- 1 cup is a baseball.

- 1 ounce (oz) of nuts is a loose handful.

- 1 teaspoon equals 1 playing die.

- 1 tablespoon is a thumb tip.

- 3ouncesz of meat equals a deck of cards.

These sizes are not accurate, but they may help a person manage their food consumption when the right tools are not accessible.

6. Eat thoughtfully: Many individuals benefit from mindful eating, which entails being completely aware of why, how, when, where, and what they consume. Making more nutritious eating choices is a direct effect of getting more in touch with the body. People who practice mindful eating also aim to eat more slowly and appreciate their meal, focusing on the flavor. Making a meal endure for 20 minutes enables the body to register all of the signals for satisfaction. It is crucial to concentrate on being content after a meal rather than full, and to keep in mind that many "all-natural" or low-fat meals are not always a good option.

People should also examine the following questions about their lunch choices:

• Is it excellent "value" for the calorie cost?

• Will it provide satiety?

• Are the components healthy?

• If it has a label, how much fat and salt does it contain?

7. Stimulus and cue control: Many social and environmental indicators may want to result in needless eating. For example, some individuals are more inclined to overeat when watching television. Others have problems delivering a dish of chocolate to someone else without stealing a piece. By being aware of what may trigger the urge to snack on empty calories, individuals might think of methods to change their routine to reduce these triggers.

8. Plan ahead: Stocking a kitchen with diet-friendly items and making regular meal plans will result in a dramatic weight reduction. People seeking to lose weight or keep it off should clean their kitchen of processed or junk foods and ensure that they have the supplies on hand to cook easy, wholesome meals. Doing this may help avoid hasty, unplanned, and irresponsible eating. Planning meal selections before coming to social gatherings or restaurants could help make the procedure smoother.

9. Seek social support: Embracing the support of loved ones is a vital aspect of a successful weight-reduction journey. Some individuals may choose to ask friends or family members to join them, while others may prefer to utilize social media to share their progress. Other routes of help may include:

• A good social network

• Group or individual counseling

• Exercise clubs or partners

• Employee help programs at work

10. Stay positive: Weight reduction is a slow process, and a person may feel disheartened if the pounds do not slip off at precisely the pace that they had expected. Some days may be tougher than others while adhering to a weight reduction or maintenance program. An effective weight-loss program demands that the person continue and not give up when self-change appears too tough. Some individuals may need to reset their objectives, possibly by lowering the overall amount of calories they are intending to consume or modifying their activity routines. The main thing is to retain a good mindset and be consistent in working toward overcoming the hurdles to healthy weight reduction. based on rules and regulations imposed by governments. Examples of such measures include eliminating UPFs from school meals, raising the price of SSBs by imposing a tax, and utilizing subsidies to decrease the price of fruit and vegetables.

CONCLUSION

None of the techniques that have been presented to promote weight loss or the maintenance of weight reduction is widely accepted as having any use in weight management. The only strategy that is universally recognized as having any utility in weight management is the clear necessity of raising energy expenditure to intake. Both the individual intervention and the data supporting the usefulness of combinations of techniques are lacking, with the findings ranging from one research study to another and with the individual. The individual intervention is inadequate in terms of its effectiveness. Recent studies that have focused on finding and researching people who have been successful in managing their weight have discovered several similar approaches that have been used by these individuals. Self-monitoring, communication with others, and support from those around you are all included in this. Participating in regular physical exercise, developing problem-solving abilities (in order to cope with challenging circumstances and situations), and developing skills to avoid relapse are all important. On the other hand, other factors that have been identified as contributing to effective weight control approaches include individual preparedness, which may be defined as a strong personal drive to achieve success in weight management.